I0438209

The Delectable Habit Of Losing Weight

How to successfully commit to your weight loss goals

Haylyn Quill
The polar bear mama

Book Design by: Polgarus Studio
Editing by: Sharon Honeycutt

Printed in the United States of America

To my readers,

Thanks for buying The Delectable Habit of Losing Weight. One key way of committing to your goal is to stay on track. As my special way of saying thanks, I'd like to give you my **free** downloadable tracking journal. Stay motivated as you track your day-to-day success with inspiring quotes from my book.

Sign up via the link below and **The Delectable Habit of Losing Weight Tracking Journal** is yours.

http://eepurl.com/cPAdcf

Stay empowered. Stay inspired.

Sincerely,

Haylyn Quill
the polar bear mama

Contents

In life, you either need inspiration or desperation.
–Tony Robbins

The Journey Begins:
What's a mama to do when fat's got her back against the wall?

First, let me say I am not a nutritionist, nor a personal trainer. I'm not a dietician or even a life coach. I'm just a woman, albeit a "super" one, who grew disgusted with the unsightly, less than "super" silhouette in the mirror and who was admittedly horrible to that image. I didn't love "her." I should have, but I didn't.

Instead, I criticized her, made her feel unworthy and undeserving. I was ashamed of her, unable to see past the stress in her sunken eyes or the dark, weary circles underneath them. I didn't stop to think about the nonstop, tedious work she did day after day to care for her family. I got mad at her instead for letting it get this bad, and I hated how she looked—like a beaten, bloated, worn-down, tore-the-hell-up woman.

Looking back, it's scary to realize I had become a bitter, self-loathing woman because I'd put on weight. But I was. I was bitter and overweight—more than forty pounds over, and it wasn't sitting pretty either.

No softly rounded romance-novel hips over here. Mine resembled a soggy box left out in the rain, all mush with a side of bumpy. And my butt? Instead of an enviable plumpness, my butt looked concave and deflated and WIDE (I'm shuddering here).

And where might, you ask, did the weight settle? It took up residence in my midsection, my face, my shoulders … you name it. I had become a woman of round proportions, a rotund (always liked that word—never thought I'd use it to describe me), misshapen version of myself … and I hated it.

To those who strive to lose hundreds, forty pounds might not seem like much. I would never downplay a daunting challenge such as that. People who overcome such odds are amazing, and I applaud their perseverance and determination. But each person's journey is different and their struggle relative. Being overweight by *that* amount—by forty pounds—shattered my self-esteem. And it showed.

I didn't feel good in my own skin and that affected all facets of my life, from intimacy to frumping (probably not a word, but I like it) around in ill-fitting clothing to hide the weight. I also began to hate taking pictures and going out—I didn't want my friends to see me. Of course, they would be kind and say encouraging things, but their words only made it worse.

Still, shirking away from the world wasn't enough for me to change what I did on a day-to-day basis. I had young kids. After taking care of all their needs and my husband's, I had nothing left to give to myself—that is until I suffered through a two-week bout of knee pain, pain that cut so deep I could barely get up the stairs in my house, pain that sent me to the office of an orthopaedic specialist.

The pain was excruciating. You should have seen me after a few steps: My face contorted into a grimace. My teeth clenched tight. My body hunched over in paralyzing pain, all because my knees were pounding and throbbing like I had muscle fatigue on top of muscle fatigue on top of muscle fatigue. I felt as if my body was turning against me, rebelling against the emotional and physical abuse I heaped on it.

Just a hot mess with bad knees.

The stairs became the bane of my existence, and my children, unfortunately (*but not so much*), became my gophers. In retrospect, I'd like to think I was doing them a favor. They needed the exercise, right? It was winter, and what better way to stay healthy and active than climbing a set of stairs—one, three, a hundred times a day?

Back to my knees. I was at the doctor, "knowing" I had the worst-case scenario. (You know … that one devastating, crippling syndrome you spent hours online researching. The one everyone else has too and it's just the worst ever with only a sliver of hope you'll make it through? I was absolutely certain I had that one.)

Turns out I didn't. Go figure! What I did have was a snarky, sarcastic-ass doctor who told me my knees looked fine but were "deconditioned." *And what does that mean, Doc?* Well, in layman terms it meant that I had forgotten about "me," and my knees were acting out like a petulant child, demanding my attention. Dr. Sarcasmo told me that I needed to take care of myself and—get this: *lose the damn weight.*

Say what?

Well, I'll tell you, I took this bit of smarts home with me that night and completely ignored it. What did he know? He wasn't a mother of four. I had real and important things to worry about. There was homework, basketball practice, T-ball sign up. A baby to feed. Not to mention the laundry, cooking, cleaning, all of which was waiting for me after the paying gig.

Take care of myself? Give me something I can use, man.

Eventually, after a few weeks of icing, heating, and sleeping on the couch, my knees got better, but my mirror didn't. The fat under my chin told a story only a chip lover could understand. And my clavicles? Those poor babies had gone missing under an avalanche of bloat. The weight was piling on, and deep down I knew that it was only a matter of time before something else gave out … or worse.

Still, I was stubborn. It would be another month before I finally licked the last remnants of sour-cream-and-onion chip residue from my fingers and said, "Enough already." Enough with feeling sluggish and looking rotund (there's my word). Enough with the same three rotating outfits day after day, hole after hole. And enough of being a critical miscreant to myself.

I was truly fed up, but there was more. In the back of my mind, I was afraid. I feared more severe health risks down the road. I feared the lack of intimacy with my partner would become permanent. And I feared my children would replicate my behaviour. Fear is what actually propelled me to act, to do something different.

To act now.

And I did.

A goal properly set is halfway reached.
-Zig Ziglar

Chapter One

Be a goal setter

The mama polar bear has one goal in mind: to survive. Each and every thing she does is in direct support of that one goal. Her survival means everything to her. She has little ones depending on her. She must ensure she is at her best so that she can be her best. Her goal is that simple.

Live.

Change is the only constant in this world, and it constantly sucks, and every once in a while, it gets to suck royally. Kicking old food habits wasn't easy. I was comfortable eating all the good stuff, and by "good stuff" I meant my kids' stuff: the cookies, the candy, and ice cream … *my goodness the ice cream*. I'm salivating just thinking about a creamy, sweet pint of raspberry and cream. Yes, I said the whole pint. A whole, decadent pint …

Wait! What was I discussing again?

Yes! Change.

I had to stop eating what my children ate, but eating what they ate had become habit. If they got a cookie, I would eat a cookie. If they ate crackers, I would have crackers. Special fast-food treats for them? Sure, a fast-food treat for me too (and it wasn't a salad). It was a habit that I took on unconsciously, one that expanded my waistline dramatically.

So first change first, I broke out of that habit—cold turkey. And since I was the food buyer, it wasn't too hard to keep it out of the house, even if that didn't please the others in the household. For about three weeks, we were a cranky, bummed-out family who gave anyone with a snack the evil eye. I had to do it though. I had to nix it all. No cookies, no ice cream, no candy, and no chips crossed our home's threshold. Yeah, they were bummed, but I let them know that if they were really that hungry, they could grab an apple and drink some water. And to show them I really meant business, I had to follow suit. (You can imagine how many apples spoiled during that time.)

They say breaking a habit is easier, in theory, if you have something new to substitute for it. So, I found a substitute.

A goal.

A life-changing goal.

My goal was simple (again, in theory at least): lose twenty-five pounds in six months. I started with twenty-five because that number wasn't fifty (I truly needed to lose fifty). Plus, I like numbers that end in five—at least I do when I'm pumping gas (Why? I haven't a clue). But even a less challenging twenty-five seemed like a fleeting thought.

After all it *was* twenty-five pounds.

Twenty-five HUGE calorie-reducing pounds.

On average, most weight loss occurs at a rate of one to two pounds a week, or so I've heard, and only if you are burning calories at a higher rate than you are eating them.

So I had to burn more than I ate, and I had to do it completely through my food intake because I had no plans to change anything else I did. I wasn't planning to join a gym or even get outside to walk more—and forget about stepping on that "step" thing in the basement. Not committed at all.

All my weight had to fall off based on my eating habits.

All twenty-five pounds of it. Gulp! Let's face it: I was having trouble losing just one, and now I was talking about swinging twenty-plus? Scary thought. And what if I failed? What if the mind was willing, but the body wasn't?

What if?

Afraid much? Yes, I was afraid. I was afraid of failing a goal of twenty-five because I'd failed before with much lower numbers. Twenty-five was a scary number, but then so was having bad knees and a bad back. So was not being able to play tag with my children in the summer. So was not being able to look at myself in the mirror without a scathing, demeaning remark. Yes, I was afraid. My weight scared me to death. My fat had my back against the wall. What was I going to do about it? Run? Hide?

Heck no! Not this time. This time I was going to get focused. Get determined. Motivated. Fear was my ally. Weight be damned. I had a goal.

Goals are foundation builders. They define and shape a journey's path. They provide a reason to take that long walk.

We set goals each day. Our daily routines are examples of this. We wake up, brush our teeth, and brew our coffee. Why should a goal to drop some pounds be any different from any other goal we set and accomplish? Why can't this goal become part of the daily routine, just as brushing your hair is? It can, and it should.

So set a goal. No matter how small the goal might be, declare it. Write it down with a big red marker and post it somewhere. Shout it to the world. Let your significant other and all your friends know you've got it. Blast it on social media.

Put it out there in the universe, and make it a concrete action item. Set one big goal or little ones along the way. What's important is to set it and then remind yourself of that goal every time temptation calls, and *boy will it shout when it does come calling.*

Ice Cream (I'm drooling again).

And remember, your goal is yours alone. Refuse to be distracted by those who tell you otherwise or seek to change your goal to one that best suits them.

Your goal is good. You do you.

We cannot solve our problems with the same thinking we used when we created them.

– Albert Einstein

Chapter Two
Change your mind

The polar bear mama knows how to eat to live. She is one of the largest, if not the largest, land-bound meat-eaters in the world. She is a survivalist, and her body is perfectly designed for and suited to live in the Arctic Circle. When she eats, she eats only to live. She does not eat out of frustration or pain or sadness or anger; she eats for her own well-being and that of her family. She doesn't eat just to eat. She eats strategically and with purpose. Her favorite meal is the seal, and when she dines, she dines on only the best of the seal, leaving the remains for scavengers to finish up. She eats what she must to ensure she is at peak performance … and that is enough.

Reprogramming the ole noggin is a big undertaking. It's a pain in the donkey tush to change how you think about something when you've been trained to think about it the wrong way from the beginning. Most people hate change. It's uncomfortable and it sucks because you have to … you know … **CHANGE**. But how many times have you heard "eat to live, not live to eat" in some discussion about weight?

It's a complete brain screw. It sounds simple enough to understand, but it isn't simple enough at all to absorb and implement.

Especially for me. You see, I had gotten used to eating crap. I did this throughout my pregnancy, and considerably more after I gave birth to my littlest person. I just ate whatever was available, and I didn't care. I was exhausted, hormonal, and just not giving a freak um cookie killer. I had a teenager, a tween, a preschooler, and a newborn. I was shot to all heck and back.

And because I didn't care and was barely functioning anyway, I ate what was quick, dirty, and tasted good. That meant cookies, candy; chips (binged on chips every day for half a year. No lie.), and ICE CREAM!!!

I ate it all and then went out and got fast food for dessert. I was living to eat—or at least to maintain the little energy I had.

So I gained weight when, typically, I should have been losing it. Now, I'm not here to beat myself up for the past. We can always look back at things in retrospect and say, "I should've done this or not done that." I had a choice, and I chose to eat poorly. It is what it is.

When I finally decided to stop and set my goal for weight loss, I had to reprogram my brain to accept the challenge. I had to stop thinking that I needed to eat when I didn't. I had to learn that more is exactly that—more to lose.

And it wasn't just about the eating. It was challenging to understand that I couldn't eat like that anymore. Forty was right around the corner, my body could no longer metabolize that kind of mindless abuse, and on top of that, I wasn't active. I wasn't a gym-goer. I barely made my walks twice a month. I sat in the house at the beck and call of my daughter and the rest of my family, managing all their needs and casting aside my own.

So, in order for me to take control of my eating I had to say no:

Do you want some candy, Mommy? No, thank you.

Do you really need those chips? Not at all!

I said no to anything and everything that put my goal in jeopardy, and I wasn't happy about it. For the first few weeks, it sucked to say no. I would say it through clenched teeth because I really wanted those chips and I really wanted that fruit snack, but I knew I didn't need any of it. I needed fruits and vegetables and water. I needed fuel for my body to live and operate effectively, not fuel to satisfy a fleeting urge.

Lucky for me, I wasn't averse to said fruits and vegetables. And equally lucky for me was the abundance of such items in my household. Believe it or not, I made sure my family ate well, even when I didn't. I'd do the healthy meal thing with them, and then after the kids were asleep, I would sit down with a big bag of chips and eat that as my "snack."

Did I need a whole freakin' bag of chips? Not at all, but I ate them anyway because I wanted to and I didn't care.

Surprisingly, it didn't take as long as I thought it would to reorganize my brain's thoughts on food. Soon, after taking a stand, I began to look at food as a source of fuel for my body. It became a tool to ensure I remained in good working order, not a source of comfort to manage my frustrations or emotions or lack of self-esteem. Fuel, like a car, is only needed when it's needed. They say, "Don't top off when refueling." Same concept here—don't top off. Eat what you need; don't overfill your tank.

It's important to rethink how food meets your needs. It cannot solve your problems, and you shouldn't try to hide behind it. We are born with an innate mental "stop" button. When we were little, our bodies recognized when we'd had enough. Unfortunately, some of us may have been retrained over time to ignore that button. We were forced to eat until *someone else* felt we were full. But what we learned can be unlearned. You have the power to retrain your brain and your body to view food in a new light. Eat to satiate your hunger, not to overindulge your appetite. Eat what you need to eat, not what you want.

Always keep your goal at the front of your mind when you are making choices about food. Embracing your goal and implementing a "no" mentality will go a long way.

Remember the end game and ask yourself, *do I need it, or do I just want it? Is what I'm about to eat truly fuel for my body, or just fuel for an urge or an emotion? Will eating this help me achieve my goal?*

If the answer is "No!" leave it and move on. You don't need it, and neither do your thighs.

Research is formalized curiosity.
It is poking and prying with a purpose.
-Zora Neale Hurston

Chapter Three
You've got homework

I'm a skeptic at heart, and I love to research facts. Anything you say, I'm like, "Hold up! Let me check that out." When it came time to research the "how to" for the twenty-five-pound-burning question, I went to my computer and typed in "How to lose weight?"

As expected, tons of *do this, no do that and try this, no try that* sites popped up. The Internet is indeed glorious. You are literally inundated with and stalked by a plethora of information that "really works."

Clicking through the diverse litany of weight-loss products and miraculous-results diets, I got sidetracked by an ad. It was an ad about … Yessss! Polar bears.

I clicked on it. (Of course, right? If not, we wouldn't be here.) I couldn't help it. Polar bears are just so darn cute, plus, I have a soft spot for animals. I ended up on a site discussing the changing diet of the polar bear. It wasn't a happy piece. It discussed how the polar bear's food source has steadily declined due to its changing environment.

Now, if you really want to tick me off, show me an animal being abused or threatened or living in captivity. I can't bear to see that. I'm not even a fan of zoos. Seeing animals caged in man-made environments, pacing around, looking morbid and hopeless upsets me. I know some zoos do wonderful things to keep animals from otherwise becoming extinct, but still, it tears me up.

But I digress. As I perused the article, I came across a captioned picture of a mother bear and her cub. In the picture, mama looked intense, focused, healthy, and solid. From her pebble-toned snout to her snowy paws, she was fierce. And I thought she has to be all of those things because she is a mama. She has to be strong and focused.

She has to be solid—not perfect, but solid and whole. If she's too thin, then she's starving; if she's too heavy, then she's not effective. She needs to be her target weight and healthy. There are predators out there who threaten her young; her health is directly related to her ability to fend them off. Her security depends on her properly fueling her body.

After reading the article and mentally cursing out all the predatory sub-humans of the world, I dug a little deeper. I looked up female polar bear diets and discovered they eat a lot of fat. I mean a lot. Good for the polar bear, not so good for me—or was it?

I kept reading. For all the fat they ate, they ate few carbohydrates. Hmm … low carb, high fat … *didn't I read about that somewhere?* I did.

And that one flashing thought began to answer my "how do I?" question.

I chose to go low carb, high fat, simply because

1. It was the best choice for *me*.
2. It met all *my* needs.

Now, here are the whys.

First, it was my best choice because, like the mama bear, I couldn't be hungry. I detest being hungry. I am a super grouch if the stomach is grumbling. It's one of the first things I even told my husband about me—our icebreaker moment. *"Make sure I'm fed."* I said. *"Or it can get ugly real quick."*

I researched and discovered that a low-carb, healthy-fat choice would be satiating. No need to snack in between meals and a fully sated feeling throughout the day. Since I've begun, I found that to be true. Sometimes I can go for a whole day on one good meal. Not one hunger pain. I've even had to remind myself at times, *"shouldn't you be eating something?"*

Being satiated conquered the temptations. All the chips, candy, and high-carb foods like pizza, I didn't need them. Did I think about them? Yes. They were part of my past life, and my mind remembered how they used to taste and what need they fulfilled. They filled a desire, a craving, but they weren't truly satiating, which is why I was also looking for more. They would always be there, but things had changed. My thoughts on food had evolved. I was using food as fuel for my body, not as fuel for an urge, so no whim eating—and plus, I was making steady progress on my goal. I didn't want to derail that.

Second, my needs were met. I absolutely loved all the foods I *could* eat. Say hello to cheeses, creams, berries, veggies, butter, and chicken. The list was endless. Anything I wanted, there was a satisfying equivalent to the unhealthy version I had scarfed down before. We're talking chocolate mint truffles and low-carb chocolate-chip cookies to die for. Addictive is an understatement when I think about these delicacies.

Just as the polar bear mama eats to stay sharp and focused for her family and herself, I wanted the same for myself and my family. This new way of eating met this need tenfold. After I began to eat low carb, healthy high fat, I gained a new sense of clarity. My memory improved. I was forgetting less, and for me that was saying something. There's truth to "mommy brain." It was fuzzy central in there for a long while.

Keeping my goal in mind, I believed I could meet my weight-loss expectations this way. And I did. During my first week, I lost five pounds. Talk about a motivation booster. Of course, I knew this was merely the beginning of my body flushing out the bad and beginning the process of accepting the new, but I liked it. I really liked it.

Now, there are different versions of eating low carb, healthy high fat. Some are more extreme, like Paleo, which restricts your carbs to less than twenty grams or something in that range. It also has something to do with ketones and ketosis. (As I said before, I'm just a mom. I haven't any real knowledge about eating the Paleo way, so don't quote me on anything. You've got to do your own research.) If I had to categorize myself, I would say I'm more of a moderate low-carbie. I eat low-carb foods in moderation, but I don't track my grams to a great extent. I just try to keep within a mental boundary of fifty to one hundred grams. Some days I eat less; other days I'm at the higher end of the spectrum.

It has never been my intention to push my body into starvation mode for weight-loss glory. Been there and done that before. (Do cayenne pepper and maple syrup sound familiar to anyone?) I like my fruits, and I like my almond butter, and I definitely like my chocolate. I eat it almost every day. I began after reading an article on a centenarian who ate a square of chocolate each day.

Sounds like good living to me.

I piggybacked off that so quickly that I had inhaled a square before I even finished reading the page. It is my sweet indulgence, and I eat the good stuff too—none of that milk-chocolate brouhaha (not that I'm judging). The higher the cocoa content, the better. For me, it's got to be rich, dark, and decadent.

So to wrap up this chapter, I can't stress enough that you need to research the "how to." Just as you probably would take the time to learn your craft through training and education, you should also train for your new lifestyle eating habit. Make it a priority to seek all the knowledge you can.

Make *your* body a priority. Treat it kindly and with respect. Don't just jump into anything that looks good. It may be right for the person in the ad, but that doesn't make it right for you no matter how often they tell you "it really works!" Make sure to take stock of the pros and cons. What are the long-term health benefits or concerns? Talk to a nutritionist and/or a doctor. Ask them what can possibly work for you.

It may even help to answer the same questions I did:

Why is it the best choice for me?

Will it fill my needs, and will it get me to my goal?

Do what you need to do to make an educated choice that works best for you.

Be a skeptic, and do your homework.

Meticulous planning will enable everything
a man does to appear spontaneous.
-Mark Caine

Chapter Four
Plan to eat. Simply.

In the wild, the polar bear mama is a planner. She prepares and anticipates the lean months ahead of time. When food is in abundance, she eats well, builds her reserves and is smart about what she consumes. Her favorite source of fuel is the seal, but she doesn't devour the entire animal; she eats only the best part—its skin and blubber—and leaves the rest.

By planning and eating only the very best of her meal, she is able to make it through the times of famine and scarcity and survive the harsh climate in which she lives. Because she plans to eat and eats simply, she has all the energy she needs to protect her young and herself.

When I first began my new lifestyle habit of eating, I "tried it on for size" for a bit. I scoured the Internet looking for recipes that fell in step with my new way of thinking, reviewing a ton of low-carb offerings. I marked the recipes I liked with a big blue star and added them to a bookmark folder titled "low-carb recipes."

Pretty simple, huh?

Once I had a pretty good number of recipes, I created my shopping list. This list would ultimately become my standard "go to" list. A list of items always on hand in the house. I've included this list at the end of this book. This list has been a life saver for me by virtually eliminating temptation and simplifying my eating. With my shelves fully stocked, everything I needed would always be close; thereby eliminating my "lazy" excuse—those times when I was too lazy to go to the store and would end up just eating whatever was in the house. Junk food!!!

My purpose behind everything I did was to alleviate the added stress that comes from trying to figure out an extensive meal to prepare and cook, especially when I was cooking only for myself. The rest of the family wasn't on board with my new lifestyle change (we'll talk more about this); they still wanted the cookies and the candy and the chips. I was alone in my journey, but that was okay because it was my goal to meet.

For the first few weeks, I made lots of new things, from main courses to side dishes to desserts. Some worked, some failed, but all the recipes were suited to the progression toward my goal, even if they turned out awful. (For the record, I suck at making low-carb fudge.)

It was a hodge-podge of sorts, but from this trial-and-error period came a small cache of easy-to-make, suitable recipes from which I could pull consistently and enjoy. A few of these recipes, I've included at the end of this book. Try them. You won't be disappointed. Another bonus was that I could make multiple servings of these meals, and because they were *sooooo* freakin' good, I didn't mind eating them more than once … and these meals had to be good. They were competing with the household chips and cookies in the cabinet above the oven.

I found a simple sense of comfort in eating the same meals consistently; it made life much easier, and I had much less worry. I knew I was coming home night after night to a delicious meal that I would immensely enjoy, kind of like a coveted writing place or an adoring husband to curl up next to … yes, like that. Plus, bulk meal planning works wonders for staying on goal and not deviating. Just a quick warm-up and you're all set.

Now, one worry I did have about my new lifestyle change was the cost. I didn't have a ton of money to throw at a grocery store cashier. I had a food budget for the family, and out of that budget, I needed to carve my own budget as well.

Remember when we talked about researching and learning your craft? Well, I made it my business to do diligent research on buying food to satisfy a low-carb/high-fat lifestyle while being on a low-dollar/high-cost-of-living budget.

At first, I browsed the websites. Then I got bored and moved on to videos.

Jackpot!

I found a ton of video information on low-carb shopping and was particularly interested in one where this hulked-up guy bought a week's worth of food for $50. And he got it from of all places …

Walmart.

Now granted, it didn't look like some of the Walmart stores I've been to (that is a book in itself), but he was making a point: shopping for my kind of food didn't have to be expensive.

I could achieve my goal with a little due diligence and some ill-fitting booty shorts (needed to gain entry to the store). In the end, I never made it to a Walmart—I couldn't find my shorts. But I did make it to a few other large chain stores that carried exactly what I needed and at a cost I could work with.

Here's the lesson: If you plan to eat simply, I believe you will find it easy to stay on track, just as I did. You will build a comfortable food schedule for yourself where you treat yourself to something delicious and filling every day, all day. Planning your meals can help you avoid going to an outside source for your fuel. I know it helped me.

You might be surprised to know that I lost the taste for dining out; I didn't want to spoil my palate for just a fleeting craving. I desired exceptional food from a top chef that was familiar to me. Myself. I would always know exactly what went into my meals—no hidden-agenda, sneaky carb overloads. And because I prepared it in advance, I didn't have to wait around after a long day of work or a stressful day with the family to have my meal.

Prudent Planning. Simple eating.

Delectable.

Remember that guy that gave up? Neither does anyone else.

– Unknown

Chapter Five
Stay the course

I am a firm believer that the naysayers, the haters, and the nonbelievers of the world have been the catalyst behind many success stories. There's no better stimulus than a doubting person or a negative thinker to light a fire under a procrastinator's pooper. Heck, this book itself was indirectly influenced by a nonbeliever.

But that is another story.

The point is I love the people who say, "I can't" or "Maybe you should do this instead." It gives me a thrill-seeking, toe-tapping, eye-twinkling rush to do the exact thing they said I couldn't do and then throw it back in their face, albeit subtly and with a "POW! That's what you get, B*&%$es!"

This chapter excites me because it addresses the obstacles that change produces.

I love my family, but they sucked sour gumballs when it came to supporting me. Here I was, cooking up a storm and testing out new foods, and they couldn't care less.

Consider a few interactions in my home:

Me: Hey honey, I got this new chicken recipe. It's so good. Try some.

Husband: Nah, I'm good.

Me: Hey sweetie. Did you notice anything different? I've lost like ten pounds. Proud of me?
Husband: Nah, I'm good.
And my favorite …
Daughter (with a screwed-up face as she watches me eat): Ewww! Mommy, that smells really bad.
Me: GO TO YOUR ROOM!

With little support in my household, I became my own support system, a one-woman cheerleading squad shouting to myself, virtual pom-poms and all, that I was a goal setter with a mission to complete.

My new lifestyle journey meant setting *myself* up for success by— get this—*meeting my needs* and *keeping my goal* at the top of my list. It was about staying the course and seeing the naysayers for what they were: propulsion ammunition.

It's quite easy to allow a lack of emotional support to derail a goal to change your lifestyle. (Again, it's about change and their resistance to it.) But if I'd allowed the nonbelievers to affect my progress, then I would have made it about them; they would have become a factor in my success, except it wasn't about them. It could never be. It was all about me.

One major way I supported myself was by taking food and drink with me whenever I left the house. Whether it was a piece of chicken breast or a cup of tea, I made sure that I would never have to search for goal-derailing sustenance outside. Being prepared eased my anxiety and eliminated a great deal of the pressure associated with managing outside forces. If temptation called, I knew I had what I needed in a baggie or in my cup to combat it.

It's an understatement to say that derailing triggers are abundant. Anything from stress to emotional trauma to that visit from Aunt Flo can hinder progress. Triggers can be anything and come from anywhere, unmercifully chipping away and taking little nicks out of your resolve. Unless you have some really good putty to continuously fill in the nicks, eventually any resolve you have will crumble under the instability.

Having said that, nothing chipped away at my resolve quicker or more effectively than stepping on the scale and seeing it go up and not down. No matter how many times I was warned against weighing myself daily, I still did it. I was impatient. I wanted to see results quickly.

Unfortunately, it doesn't work that way, and I was setting myself up for disappointment with unrealistic expectations. So many factors affect weight, and women are very effective at holding onto it. Just like the mama polar bear, our bodies are built for survival—the survival of our species. We are water hoarders and storage units for fat. And while each of us is probably aware of our weight fluctuations during certain times of the month, it still sucks to see this evidence staring back at us like a sneering antagonist. One minute you've dropped two and then the next minute you're up by three—a disheartening motivation killer to say the least.

It was especially during these times that I had to continue staying the course and really focus on eating well. I chose not to give in to hormonal cravings while still being kind to myself as I should. I looked upon that time as my "time-out" period. No scale, no scrutiny.

Staying the course isn't about perfect progression. It's about making steady, focused headway toward your goal. It's about recognizing your triggers for what they are—the naysayers, the haters, the chippers—and managing them. It's about treating yourself with respect and giving yourself the time your body needs to go through its natural processes without scrutiny.

It's about patience and awareness. Be your own cheerleader. Throw shade to the naysayers. Commit to yourself and stay the course.

If you can't measure it, you can't improve it.

– Peter Drucker

Chapter Six
Track It

O ne thing about a goal is that it tends to look, for the most part, like the finish line at the end of a marathon, impossible to see until you're on the last leg of the journey. Now, I've never run a marathon, but I do know that alongside that long, thigh-jarring road are markers that track how far you've come and how far you have to go.

These markers are just as important to the runners as the pep-rally folks who shove water into their sweaty palms. The markers let them know they are closer now than they were before and to stay the course.

These powerful and motivating tracking tools keep the spirited and the weary connected to their goal, which is the finish line.

Over the years, I've accumulated my share of semi-success and failure stories regarding my weight, and the beginning of each is the same. I dive right in with gusto and fervor, believing this time around (*for real, for real*) will be different. I post little "positive thought" sticky notes around the house and print out motivating quotes and tape them to the fridge. As suggested, I buy new sneakers because today is the first day of walking my way to a "new me."

Initially, these worked. For the first few weeks, I was in it to win it. Nothing could stop me—and nothing did—except that I did *nothing* after those initial weeks, which I guess is actually something.

The thing was I kept doing the same things over and over, expecting a different result, a result I was never going to get. It wasn't until I looked at new ways to keep my motivation alive and thriving that I changed my course of action.

Now, I don't know about you, but money is a pretty powerful motivator for me. It's not the end-all be-all, but I'll be damned if I'll pass up an opportunity to be paid for something I'm already doing. So when my husband's company sent me a brochure flaunting a $350 incentive to join their wellness program, I didn't have to be told twice.

I was on it like a fly to poop, trying to figure out how to get my $350 as fast as I could by doing the least amount of work. If you aren't aware of what a wellness program is, it is essentially an incentive-driven program that is set up as a tool to aid individuals with improving their health and/or fitness.

Surprisingly, after a few weeks, I began to see the benefit—beyond the monetary incentive—of joining a wellness program. (Oh! So that's why they say, "Keep an open mind"!)

After setting up my account and profile (easy-peasy), I started tracking my weight and my eating habits on a daily basis. And yes, my eating habits were already well defined and progressing along, but the program enabled me to tangibly track them. It went from a running virtual tab in my head to a concrete, running tally on paper. And once I saw how well I was doing, inputting my day-to-day activities online, I was motivated to "keep up the good work."

I know we can't all join a wellness program through an employer, but there are so many tracking tools online that provide goal setters with program ideas or simple templates to input and track your progress. It doesn't have to be as fancy-pants as a company-designed wellness program; it can be as simple as a pretty notebook in which you track what you eat on a daily basis, jot down notes on how you feel, and track your weight.

Speaking of weight again, I would like to take a moment to talk more about tracking it. There are many opinions out there on how to do it. Should you step on a scale once a day? Once a week? Once a month? Never?

Initially, I *was* a once-a-day scale hopper, tracking and recording it in my wellness profile daily. For me, this type of tracking did more harm than good. It created a bit of anxiety in me, and I started fretting and overanalyzing the numbers on the scale.

It took a few weeks before I realized how neurotic I had become. I had begun to weigh myself three or more times a day just to see if I lost a few ounces, and if I didn't, I would try to manipulate the scale to give me the reading I wanted.

I would do things like hold onto the towel bar, stand slightly off the scale, or even place the scale in different areas of the house. I believed that the evenness of the floor (i.e., wood vs. tile) made a difference. I drove myself mad and all for a few ounces.

After a month or so of allowing a piece of digitized glass to drive me emotionally loco, I learned to say "no!" to the scale.

I stopped the daily weigh-ins and went down to once a week. I also forced myself to stop viewing my weight emotionally. Once I took the emotion out of it, weight became just a representation of force and gravity to me. I was just a mass, and weight was simply the amount of force gravity exerted on it.

When I quantified it that way, I was able to focus more on how I was feeling. Did I feel good? Did I feel focused? Did I look healthier? Did my clothes fit better? If the answers were "yes," then I was on target.

So while it is important to track your weight consistently, it is equally important to not go bonkers over what you see on the scale.

And tracking isn't just about a program or a piece of paper. One of the best ways I've found to track progress is to take note of the changes in an obscure body part over time.

(Here is where I thank my GFF K.B. because she swears by this body part.)

For me, it was my clavicles—those two horizontal bones that run between your breastbone and your shoulders. At my heaviest, my clavicles were barely visible beneath my skin, like two little blips on a screen. Maybe there, maybe not. As my weight dropped, my clavicles became more pronounced. I could actually see them as two jutting straightaways converging toward the hollow of my neck.

I continue to use these as my main progression gauge, taking note of them each morning in the mirror. It's taken a bit of time, but I do enjoy looking at them now.

It's all in the spirit of tracking your progress. Whether you choose the fat on your back or a pudgy ankle, use that as a gauge to inspire you—and love that back fat in the process. OWWWNNN IT! It's your back fat. And as you track its transformation, be kind to it even as you tell it to move the "hell" on.

Remember that tracking is a good way to stay focused. It provides you with tiny markers to remind you that you've come this far and you need to keep going. We all hope to eventually see the red ribbon at the finish line, but in the meantime, love each step of the journey.

As any mama polar bear will tell you … while you are thankful to have those maddening, but precious days with your cubs, secretly, you're thrilled to know that you'll never have to have that crazy day again.

Track it, baby, and roam on!

For every disciplined effort, there is a multiple reward.
-Jim Rohn

Chapter Seven
Reward Yourself. All the time.

L ove, love, love this chapter. It's all about paying yourself back. Yes! Abundant rewards are yours.

And it's simple, really. Treat yourself well ALL the time. Your new lifestyle isn't meant to be torturous. If it was, why the heck would you stay the course? I'm not saying it shouldn't take hard work to achieve your goals, but life is short—the only guarantee you have on this earth is that you will die. That's it. Everything else is ultimately a crapshoot.

Knowing this, the last thing I want is to be on my death bed with only a sprig of a damn sprout and a glass of crummy lemon water in my gut. When they cut me open, I want them to say, "Damn! This woman ate well."

Yes, I'm exaggerating, but my point is that changing how you eat doesn't mean you have to "change" how you eat. Food should be satisfying and yummy to the tummy. For me that included cookies, mousse, rice pudding and ... say it!

ICE CREAM!! (Trumpets sound off!)

Throughout the polar bear mama's lifetime, she will face some harsh winters when food isn't in abundance. During these times, she goes into survival mode and eats anything from reindeer to rodents to birds. During famine, she's an unapologetic opportunist that eats what she must. Why? She's got her little cubs to protect.

But there are also times when the getting is good, when food is in abundance and all that is required is a little patience and the swipe of a skilled paw. During these times she feasts on her favorites … and boy, does she feast.

Now, I can't tell you which way to go on this one, but I will tell you I'm not one to live my life in a perpetual state of famine. I want to feast like the polar bear mama feasts. I want the good stuff. Anyone for eating a blubbery, fatty seal?

I like to reward myself … all the (bleeping) time.

I eat chocolate, mousse, apple pie, berry-cheesecake smoothies, and even red-velvet truffles. The difference is, when I'm eating these delectable goodies, I know what's in them and I know that what I'm eating directly supports me in achieving my goal.

Through my research, I found all sorts of tasty ways to feed my desire for sweet, gooey treats. You've heard others say, "There's an app for that," right? Well, "There's a recipe for that." The Internet is spilling over with recipes for low-carb desserts. I've learned to make everything from cherry cobbler to crème brulee, and all of it is … *shhh … low carb.*

How sweet is that? Literally!

So that's it. Eat and eat well. Don't deprive yourself of what you want; just ensure that what you want benefits your goal progression. Do a little research, and learn how to make the things that will linger decadently on the palette.

Speaking of decadence, I found an amazing low-carb almond-butter chocolate-chip-cookie recipe online. These cookies are addictively good and ridiculously easy to make, even for a certified "non-baker" like myself. I'll include the website at the end of this book. Try them even if you aren't a low-carbie. I'm telling you, you won't be sorry.

If you aren't into baking, then find simple ways that don't require an oven to reward yourself. One of my favorite treats is simply a goblet (yes, I get fancy) full of low-carb berries covered in heavy cream with dark-chocolate chips sprinkled on top. It's a quick, simple, and *oh-so-enjoyable* treat.

The rewards don't have to be edible either. This is all about rewarding yourself your way. Heck, buy yourself a pretty new pair of underwear for every five you lose. Or if you're into coloring, a new colored pencil.

Whatever it is, reward yourself ALL the time. It will keep you motivated and looking forward to the next marker on your journey.

Motivation is what gets you started. Habit is what keeps you going.
-Jim Rohn

Chapter Eight
Make it a delectable habit

This is a short-and-sweet chapter about starting a habit and being all about it. You may have noticed throughout this book that I never referred to my goal as a "diet." There's a reason for that. For me, my weight-loss journey wasn't a diet. It was a lifestyle change. I changed my eating lifestyle, and in doing so, I created a new lifelong habit.

According to science, it takes on average sixty-six days to break a habit. Some habits can be broken in as little as eighteen days, while some take almost a year.

Do, I believe this? Yeah. It sounds about right, but who knows. What I do believe in is myself. And my self tells me that I will never go back to eating the way I did before. I've no longer the urge, nor do I see any benefit to eating as I once did.

I mentioned earlier in the book that breaking a habit and creating a new one go hand in hand. It's much easier to break a bad habit if you have a new habit to take over. But what happens after? *How do you stay with your new habit?* You stay with it by providing it with powerful, self-sustaining motivation.

So, what's my motivation?

Pure, delectable decadence. I absolutely, positively love my food. Love it. And yes, I enjoyed what I ate before, but it doesn't hold a candle to what I eat now. I'm not giving this up.

Don't get me wrong, I gave up some decent-tasting foods—I had to. And I'm perfectly okay with that because in addition to giving up those good-tasting foods, I also gave up overall bad eating, unhealthy food choices, and a gut-bloating habit. With loss, though, there should be some gains. So what did I gain? Self-love …

(Did your mind just go there, or was it just mine?)

Anyway, I gained self-love, clarity of mind, a new perspective, and a better relationship with food, which is forever evolving, continually progressing and growing in new, exciting ways. I'm excited about eating now because I know it doesn't control me. I can truly enjoy my meals and my treats and feel really good afterwards. It's a great feeling to have lost the guilt associated with food. Overall it is a win for me.

I won't go back, and I implore you not to go back either once you decide to change your eating lifestyle. Find all the reasons to stay true to the new you. Change isn't easy, but neither is stepping on a scale with fear clawing at your heart. I'll take the change any day before that lifelong anxiety.

Remember, polar bear mamas don't live to diet; we live to try it.

Start a new, delectable habit, and be habitual about it.

All you need is the plan, the road map,
and the courage to press on to your destination.
-Earl Nightingale

The Journey Continues …

The mama polar bear knows that the road is hardly paved in warm, downy grass. It's most often a treacherous, ice-packed trek filled with cold, hungry days with nothing more than the fur on her back and her cubs by her side. But it's during those times when she is at her strongest. She is her best self. She makes no excuses, and she faces any obstacle head-on.

There are no shortcuts in life. That's one line that's rung true for me each day I live. The work has to be done, and the earned reward mostly correlates to the amount of work put in.

It took me just a little under three months to drop fifty pounds.

Yes! I said *fifty in less than three months*. I lost double the weight in a little over half the time.

My lifestyle habit is no joke.

I surpassed my goal by 200 percent, and I am unbelievably excited about my new weight. I weigh less than I did prior to having my first little person, and I did this all by following through on my principles and staying true to my purpose.

After dropping fifty, I had lunch with one of my closest girlfriends. She asked me if I planned to "let up" on my eating habits now that I'd lost the weight and if I would be incorporating old foods into my new plan.

"Of course not!" I told her. "Those foods are history."

And it's true. The food I used to eat is my past, and there's no use looking back unless I'm planning to go back there, which I'm not. I now eat within the endless boundaries of my new lifestyle. I am mindful of what goes into my body. It has become second nature.

I also told her, "I don't do diets. I do habits, so why change an insanely good habit when it's serving a great purpose in my life?"

This journey is a lifelong one. I'm still progressing. I created a new goal, and I'm working on that one now. I'm not sure where I will finally end up on the scale weight-wise. I would love to be in the low 130s, but realistically that may never happen. Genetics probably won't allow it. I have meat on my thighs and hips. I've got a butt and boobs. I don't believe that my body is meant to slim down to that level anymore, and I'm okay with that. My hubby is too. Somewhere along the line though, I'm guessing I will probably peak at a threshold weight with a little extra padding left over to help keep me comfortable on those long days sitting at my computer and writing.

My body has *lived*. It's gone through many changes. It's given birth multiple times and survived decades of unrelenting gravity. The perk is gone, and I'm okay with that because I was never seeking perfection. I just wanted to feel good in my skin, look good in my clothing, and take a couple "Dang! You look good girl!" twirls in front of the mirror—which I do now. My mirror is back in my good graces, and there's love there again.

This is just the beginning. I plan to have more fun in front of my mirror, and you can as well. Commit to yourself every day and make it happen. Set your goals. Take the time to learn and find what works best for you, and follow through on that. Ignore the haters. They are only there to steal your glory. Stay motivated, and be good to yourself. Be habitual about your new lifestyle habit, and enjoy the journey.

This is all about you. Remember that. You deserve the time to indulge yourself and cater to all your needs and wants.

Remember who you are.
You are the prodigious woman.
You are the polar bear mama.
So, growl on, mama!
Growl on!

Here are a few of my regular rotation recipes with pictures I took myself. They are super quick and easy to make. Try them and see for yourself.

Warm Tuna Salad over greens

Here's a nice low-carb twist on tuna. Perfect for lunch or a quick dinner when you're tired or low on time.

Ingredients:

1 Can	Tuna Fish (I prefer packed in oil)
½ Tbsp.	Capers
¼ Cup	Heavy Whipping Cream
1 Handful	Sliced Leek or Chopped Scallions (Can do a combo of both)
1 Squeeze	Dijon Mustard (approx. 1Tbls.)
1 Pinch	Sea Salt
1 Pinch	Coarse Pepper
1 Pinch	Cayenne Pepper
1 Heavy Sprinkle	Favorite Cheese (I prefer crumbled feta or shredded parmesan)
1 Salad Plate Full	Choice of Lettuce (Romaine is my go-to)
1 Splash	Concentrated Lemon Juice

Directions:

Heat a pan over med heat. Drain tuna, but not all the way. Reserve some of the oil to coat the pan (if using non-oil-based tuna, add 1 tsp. coconut oil or a sliver of butter to pan). Dump tuna into pan along with the leeks/scallions. Stirring intermittently, cook until the leeks begin to look a bit wimpy (about 3-4 minutes). Stir in capers, mustard, salt/pepper and cayenne pepper. Cook for another minute.

Add in heavy cream, stir, and cook one minute more. Remove pan from heat. Place warm tuna on top of greens. Sprinkle with cheese. Splash with lemon juice. 1-2 servings. Enjoy!

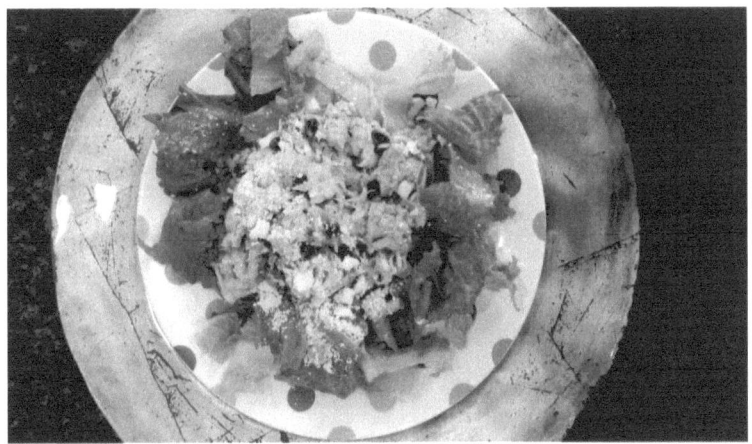

Sautéed Buttered Broccoli & Cauliflower with Blue Cheese Dressing

This simple, lovely, low-carb dish takes about six minutes to prepare. It's great as a side or on its own if you're feeling particularly veggie-licious. I personally like to pair it with a Cajun-style tuna steak.

Ingredients:

1 Steam Bag	Broccoli/Cauliflower
1 Sliver (1/2 oz.)	Butter
¼ cup (about a handful)	Thinly Sliced Leek
1 Pinch	Sea Salt/Pepper
1 Tbsp.	Blue Cheese Dressing
1 Heavy Sprinkle	Blue Cheese Crumbles (Optional)
½ Tsp.	Chopped Garlic

Directions:

Steam bag of broccoli/cauliflower according to the bag directions. Meanwhile, heat a pan on med/high and drop in butter to melt. Add in the garlic and leeks to soften and brown. Add fully steamed broccoli/cauliflower mixture to pan. Add in salt/pepper. Cook until nicely brown and semi-wilted. Add blue cheese dressing and cook about a minute more. Transfer to a plate and sprinkle with blue cheese crumbles. 2-3 Servings.

Inspired by: www.dietdoctor.com

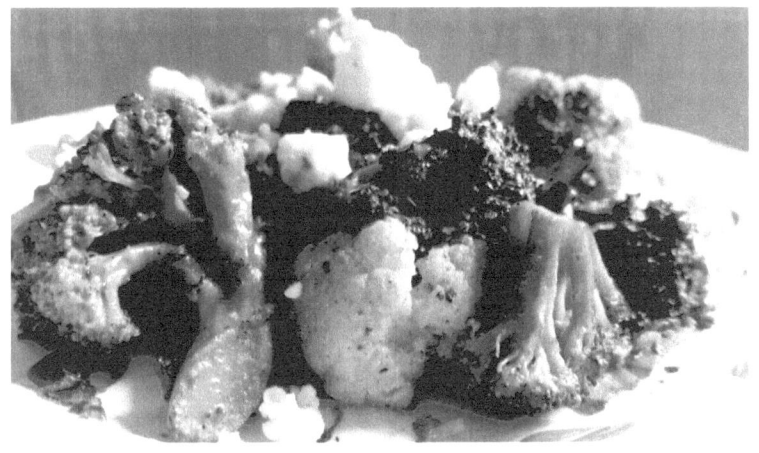

Very Merry, Very Berry Cheesecake Smoothie

This smoothie not only looks pretty, it tastes pretty too. Sweet!

Ingredients:

4-5 Fresh	Raspberries
2-3 Fresh	Strawberries (trimmed and sliced)
4-5 Fresh	Blackberries
1 Splash	Heavy Whipping Cream
1 capful	Vanilla Extract
1 oz.	Cream Cheese
1 Heaping Spoonful	Ricotta Cheese (optional but ups cheesecake factor)
8 oz.	Almond Milk (I prefer unsweetened vanilla)
4-5	Ice Cubes
2-4 Packets	Favorite Natural Low-Carb Sweetener (1 packet = approx. 2 Tsp)

Directions:

Drop all ingredients into a blender or bullet. Start with two packets of sweetener. Blend on high for about a minute or more, depending on your blender's instructions. Add in additional packets of sweetener according to your sweetness preference. 1-2 servings.

Note: Go easy on the ice as it tends to water down the creaminess of the smoothie. Start with a few and add more as needed.

Sweet variation: Use Mascarpone cheese in place of Ricotta.

Inspired by: www.the-lowcarb-diet.com

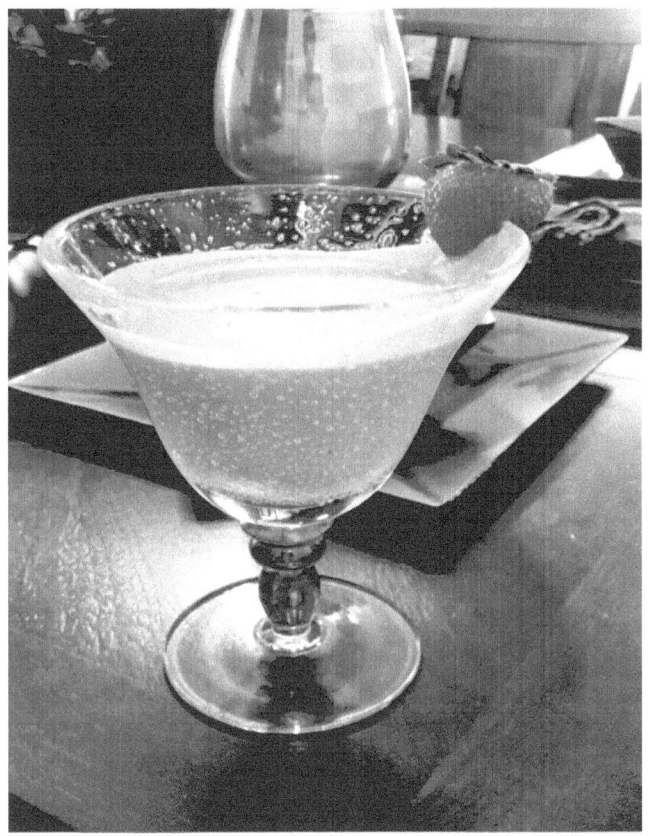

The Shopping List

A low-carb, high-fat lifestyle includes lots of veggies, lean meats, and healthy fats. This list is my "go-to" list. I keep everything on here on hand at home—always.

Almond Butter
Almond Milk
Avocado
Butter
Broccoli
Caesar Dressing
Cauliflower (Great for rice)
Chicken (Boneless/skinless thighs)
Coconut Oil
Dark Chocolate – 70% or Better Cocoa (Chips/Bars)
Eggs
Feta Cheese
Heavy Whipping Cream
Kale
Leeks
Romaine Lettuce

Scallions
Strawberries
Salmon
Sugar (i.e., Stevia/Erythritol)
Tuna (Can/steaks)
Vanilla Extract

About Haylyn Quill

Haylyn Quill the polar bear mama is a writer, mother and wife. Her passions lie in the mundane as well as the eccentric. She strives to inspire in others the motivation and drive to become their best selves. Her life, as she describes it, is a randomness of chaotic pieces concealed under a guise of predictable organization. The Delectable Habit is her first published work. Currently, she resides in New York with hubby bear and their four cubs.

Connect with the polar bear mama:
F: https://www.facebook.com/HaylynQuill/
T: https://twitter.com/polar_bear_ma

More books coming soon. Sign up to be the first to hear about new releases, giveaways and pre-release dates.
Come for the quirks, stay for the laughter.

www.thepolarbearmama.com

Courage is what it takes to stand up and speak; courage is also what it takes to sit down and listen. -Winston Churchill

Thank you for reading my book. As an indie author, reviews are invaluable. If you enjoyed the book, please consider leaving a review for it. Your kind words and constructive feedback are appreciated.
Thank You.

Dedication/Thank You

This book is dedicated to the polar bear mamas of the world. Remember who you are and what you can be. Stay inspired.

Growl on!

My deepest thanks to my family and all my friends who support me with their words, actions and understanding. Your names fill my book of gratitude.

And to all of those who were a part of this book journey. Thank you.

As promised.

Flourless Almond-Butter Chocolate-Chip Cookies
www.theviewfromgreatisland.com